Get In Shape

with Resistance Band Training

The 30 Best Resistance Band Workouts and
Exercises That Will Sculpt And Tone Your Body At Home

Want To Get In Shape Faster?
Add These Books To Your Daily Workout Routine!

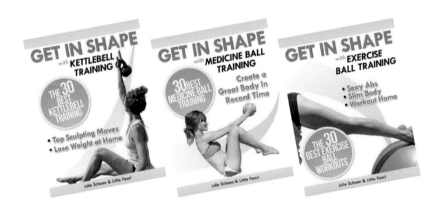

Discover Other Great Books By
Julie Schoen

Disclaimer

This book contains general information and is for informational purposes only. You should use proper discretion, and consult with a health care practitioner, before following any of the exercises, techniques, or plans described in this book. The author and publisher expressly disclaim responsibility for any adverse effects that may result from the use or application of the information contained in this book.

Contents:

Get In Shape   5

3 Effective Workout Plans   6

    10 Minute Workout Plan   8

    20 Minute Workout Plan   8

    30 Minute Workout Plan   8

The 30 Best Resistance Band Exercises   11

Exercise Index   43

Bonus Workout Soundtracks   45

GET IN SHAPE

As a woman, it seems like being envious comes with the territory. And now with the advent of social media, A-Lister celebrities, supermodels, and flawless fitness fiends flash before our eyes with the tap of a finger. Ever since I remember receiving my first "girly" magazine as a teenager, I recall that instead of obsessing over the latest make-up tips, the hottest designer labels, and trendiest hairstyles, I went immediately to the question, "What do they do to look like that?"

Put In The Work

Long, sculpted legs, flat tummies, lean arms, and backs that make men want you to walk away, there are plenty of enviable women running amuck in the world today. But rather than get jealous, which I most certainly could, I look at these gorgeous women as a source of inspiration and strength.

Most of the killer bodies owned by supermodels and celebrities don't just appear out of thin air; those women put in hours upon hours of intense training and loads of sweat. They are willing to get up at the crack of dawn, work out, and then squeeze in even more training sessions throughout the day.

And while most of us can't commit eight-hours a day to working out (and even if I could, would I?), we can, thankfully, learn from the celebrities, seeing what training methods work best and which exercises have the biggest impact in the shortest amount of time.

Getting In Shape No Longer Means Joining A Gym

Praise the lord that getting in shape no longer means buying a pricey gym membership and suffering through the grunts and projectile sweat from the nearby muscle! No, today women can get in shape in the comfort of their own home, or even take their workout outdoors, which means no more fighting over equipment, no more long drives to the gym, and, hallelujah, no more public restrooms.

Why I Love Resistance Bands

One of the most popular at-home workouts that have been a mainstay in the celebosphere for some time now is resistance bands. Inexpensive and highly effective, celebrities like Stacy Keibler, Elsa Pataky, Olivia Munn, Lauren Conrad, Elisabeth Rohm, Kelly Rowland, and La La Anthony all have been caught training with resistance bands in recent months.

Professional trainers love resistance bands because of their portability, but most of all they offer endless possibilities. Literally every muscle of your body can be worked with resistance bands and the intensity levels can be easily altered without having to purchase new equipment. This means that even if your body is totally imbalanced with super strong legs and cooked spaghetti-like arms, the same band can be used to challenge your lower body while also building strength in the upper. And because of the angles that resistance bands can provide (literally hundreds), they are able to work muscles in range of motions that would be difficult if not impossible with other types of equipment.

From Pilates instructors to professional trainers, models, celebrities, and fitness gurus, everyone loves resistance bands. Throw them in your purse or travel bag, and you don't even know they're there. And for those of us who live in small spaces, bands mean that our living rooms don't have to look like a gym in order for us to get a thorough workout at home.

So whatever your fitness goals might be – lose a few pounds, tone your legs, perk up your butt, or just feel confident in your favorite outfit – you can be sure that if it works for the women who get paid to look good, it will work for you!

Have Fun and Get Ready To Get In Shape!

3 EFFECTIVE WORKOUT PLANS

No matter what your day looks like, I know that you can find the time to squeeze in a 10-minute workout. Even in just 10 minutes, 5 times a week you will start to see incredible results. If you have more time, you can be sure that the body you will have in just a matter of weeks will be worth a little less sleep or a missed episode of Duck Dynasty.

The Equipment

Two quality resistance bands are all you will need – one flat and one tube with handles. Although similar, the two different types are used for different exercises and are hard to interchange. Speaking from experience, the tube-kind tends to be a pain if you try to place them on your feet since they will constantly roll off and snap you in the face. There are different types available and some are definitely better than others. Don't go for the cheapest brand as they tend to be made from material that wears and stretches quickly. Expect to pay around $15 - $20 for the handled tube band and $10 - $15 for the flat.

Storing the bands is simple – toss wherever! But be sure to not leave them in direct sunlight or outdoors for too long because they will start to turn brittle and may even crack and break.

Intensity

Some brands of resistance bands offer varying levels of intensity. While you can choose whichever intensity you think you'll be most comfortable with (or be like me and just choose your favorite color), know that it is fairly simple to adjust the intensity.

To change the intensity of flat bands, simply step or hold the band in a different spot. The tube bands with handles can be modified by tying a knot further down the end to stop the handle from going all the way down – this is great for modifying for shorter height as well as strength. You will find, however, that each exercise will require different lengths of bands. For example, a much longer band will be necessary if you need to step on the band while bringing your arms all the way over your head. For this reason, although it's possible to tie and untie knots during your workout, it's most convenient to have a few bands ready to go – a flat, a long tube with handles, and a modified, shorter tube with handles works best for me.

If you are losing sleep over which band intensity to choose, go with the medium or hard – you're stronger than you think you are!

10 Minute Workout

Begin by warming up with a few minutes of intense cardio, such as running sprints, jumping rope, or mountain climbers. Choose 3 band exercises, doing 1 set of 30 to 40 reps of each exercise on one side. Then do the same exercises with the same amount of reps on the other side. Try to rest as little as possible between exercises.

20 Minute Workout

Choose 6 different band exercises, doing 3 sets of 12 reps of each exercise. If the exercise is only done on one side, do 6 reps on each side to finish 1 set. In between sets, rest for 30 seconds before moving to the next exercise.

30 Minute Workout

Choose 8 different band exercises, doing 2 sets of 12 to 16 reps of each exercise. If the exercise is only done on one side, do 6 to 8 reps on each side to finish 1 set. Do 1 set of all of the exercises and take a 2 to 3 minute rest before repeating the exercises in the same order for the second set.

Insider Tips For Anchoring

When performing many resistance band exercises it is necessary for you to anchor the band, which can seem confusing or a pain in the butt at first. Have no fear! Here are some secrets for getting the most out of your resistance band workouts:

When using the tube band with handles, it's simple to anchor by placing one end of the tube with handles over the top of a door. By closing the door you will have successfully anchored your band.

To increase the intensity for certain exercises place both ends of the tube with handles over the top of the door. Shut the door and grip the center of the tube to perform your exercises.

If the exercise requires you to anchor the band but keep both handles free for you to use, you can take a spare tube band (or something similar), tie it in a small loop with a large knot, secure the knot over the top of the door, and close the door. The loop should hang over the top of the door so that you can place your resistance tube through the loop, having it anchored with both handles free.

Exercising outside will give you more options for anchoring the band, especially if there are nearby trees or fences. Some exercises work better when the band can be anchored at shoulder or hip-height.

The easiest anchor, however, is always a friend. So if you have the ability to work-out with a friend – do it! And remember, they're more than just a convenient way to secure your band; they're great motivators too!

THE 30 BEST RESISTANCE BAND EXERCISES

Each exercise lists the ideal resistance band to use (Tube with Handles or Flat) as well as the muscle groups that are targeted. Many of the exercises can be performed with either band, but be aware that when using the tube band, especially around the feet, there is a chance that it will roll off and could possibly injure you.

Also be sure that whatever you are anchoring the band to is secure so as to avoid any serious injuries that could result from an object falling on top of you.

Using resistance bands can take a few times to get used to, so be patient. After a bit of trial and error you will discover the best ways to use the bands for each exercise so as to best adapt to your body's specific needs. And believe me, the results you get from these workouts will be well worth a few minutes spent here and there tying knots or bribing a friend (or a kid) to hold the bands in place.

Get creative, have fun, and get ready to look awesome!

1. Side Reach

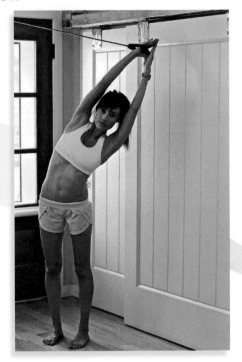

Resistance Band: Tube with Handles
Targets: Shoulders, Triceps, Biceps, and Core

Anchor the band at head-height or higher, doubling the band to increase intensity if necessary. Stand with your feet about shoulder-width apart, holding onto the band with both hands. Bring your palms together and reach your arms up straight by your ears. Keeping your feet still, lean to the side until you feel the muscles of your core starting to work. Slowly bring yourself back up to standing position.

Do all of your reps on one side before switching sides to finish a set.

2. Squat Press

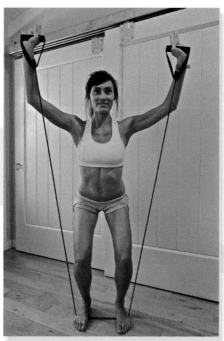

Resistance Band: Tube with Handles
Targets: Legs, Glutes, and Shoulders

Stand on the center of your band with feet about hip-width apart. Grab onto the handles, one in each hand, palms face forward. Bend your elbows and come into a squat. As you squat make sure you keep the weight in your heels and your knees and your shins far enough back that you can see your toes. Reach your arms as far above your head as possible, adjusting resistance as necessary. Lower your arms back down to your sides as you come out of the squat.

Come back to a standing position to finish 1 rep.

3. All-Fours Donkey Kick

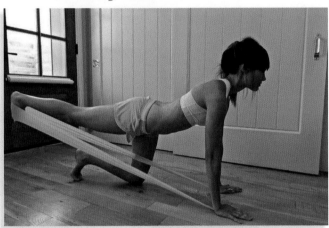

Resistance Band: Flat
Targets: Glutes

Come on to all fours. Place the center of the band over the sole of your right foot, holding on to the ends of the band with the palm of each hand. Your hands should be directly under your shoulders. Start to extend the right leg straight back, lifting the knee and the foot off of the ground. If possible, keep the lifted leg even with the ground. Make sure you press through your hands enough so that you don't sink into the shoulders. Return to the starting position.

Do all of your reps on one side before switching sides to finish 1 set.

4. Band Wrap Push-Up

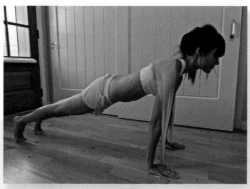

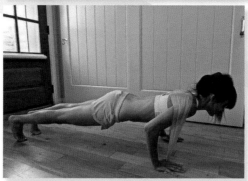

Resistance Band: Flat
Targets: Chest, Triceps, and Core

Come to the top of a push-up (plank position) with the band over your upper back and shoulder blades. Place your hands under your shoulders, holding on to the ends of the strap. The band should be taut with your arms straight. Keep the body straight as you start to bend your elbows and lower your chest down to the ground. Continue to look slightly forward as you lower. Press yourself back up to the starting position to finish 1 rep.

Until you build more strength, feel free to do as many reps as needed with your knees down on the ground.

5. Rowing Roll

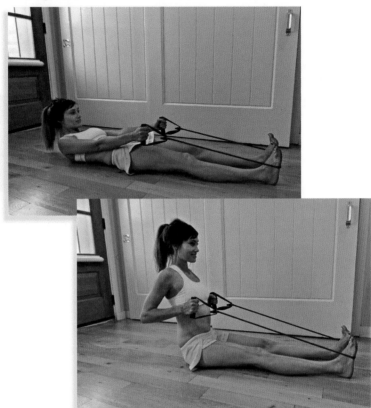

Resistance Band: Tube with Handles
Targets: Core, Back, and Biceps

Sit with your legs extended straight out in front of you. Place the tube over your feet and grab the handles, one in each hand. With the arms straight, slowly begin to roll down until just your shoulders touch the ground. It's important to do this slowly in order to work the core. Be sure that your feet stay on the ground as well. As you slowly roll back up to sit. Bend the elbows and pull the tube until your hands are at your chest and elbows are in line with your shoulders.

Straighten the arms to return to the starting position and finish 1 rep.

6. Open Close

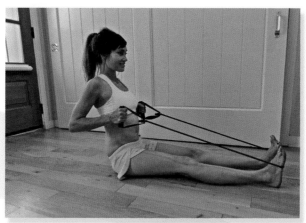

Resistance Band: Flat
Targets: Glutes and Legs

Lie on your back with your legs extended straight into the air, feet together. Place the band over the soles of your feet and hold onto each end with your hands. Begin to move your legs away from each other, bringing them into a "V" shape. You should feel resistance as you do this.

Return your legs to the starting position to finish 1 rep.

7. Boxer

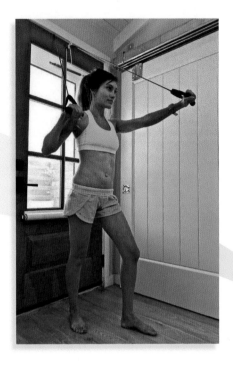

Resistance Band: Tube with Handles
Targets: Shoulders, Back, and Triceps

Anchor the center of your tube band behind you. Place your hands through each handle, standing a foot or two away from the anchor. Bring the handles to shoulder height and stagger your feet one in front of the other, front knee slightly bent. Keeping your elbows wide and away from your body, punch with one hand then the other.

Hop switch your feet and punch both hands again to complete 1 rep.

8. Triceps Raise

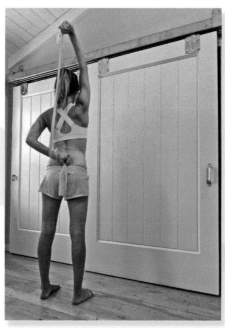

Resistance Band: Flat
Targets: Triceps

Hold the band behind your back, one end in each hand. Bring your left hand to the center of your low back and your right hand behind your head with the elbow bent. Keeping the left hand still, begin to straighten the right arm overhead. As you extend your arm, be sure to keep it close to your ear. Bend the elbow slowly to return to the starting position.

Do all of your reps on one side before switching sides to complete 1 set.

9. Rows

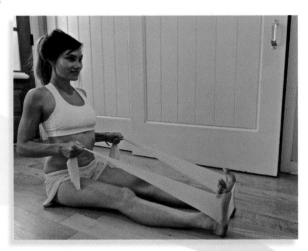

Resistance Band: Flat
Targets: Biceps and Back

Sit on the ground with your legs extended straight out in front of you. Place the band over your feet, holding one end in each hand. With the arms extended straight in front the band should be taut. Continue to sit tall as you pull the band back, bending the elbows. Pull the band back so that your hands touch or almost touch your torso -- keep the elbows near the body and squeeze the shoulder blades together.

With control, slowly return to the starting position and finish 1 rep.

10. High Low Pull

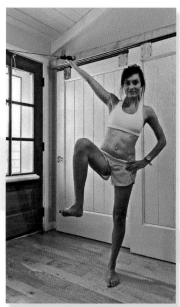

Resistance Band: Tube with Handles
Targets: Biceps, Glutes, and Core

Secure one end of the tube at door-height or higher. Stand with your feet shoulder-width apart, your right side facing the anchor. Grab onto the handle with your right hand, arm extended straight, and palm facing up. With your left hand on your hip, transfer your weight and lift the right foot off of the ground. Bend your knee and lift the foot as high as possible. As you lower your right foot back to the ground, bend your right elbow and pull the tube towards your shoulder.

Return to the starting position to complete 1 rep. Do all of your reps on one side before switching sides to finish 1 set.

11. Karate Kid

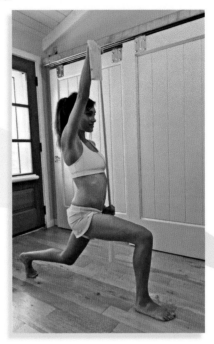

Resistance Band: Flat
Targets: Legs, Back, and Shoulders

Hold the band at chest height. The band should be taut when your hands are shoulder-width apart. Stand with your feet staggered, right foot in front of the left. Bend your knees and come into lunge. As you lunge, extend your right arm straight overhead, bicep by ear, as you pull your left arm straight down in front of your left hip. When you lunge, be sure your front knee stays over your ankle and that you are going low enough to make your front thigh parallel with the ground.

Slowly bring yourself back to the starting position. Do all of your reps on one side before switching sides to complete 1 set.

12. Overhead Press

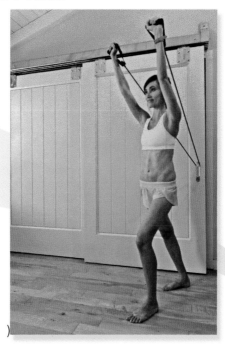

Resistance Band: Tube with Handles
Targets: Shoulders

Secure the center of the resistance band at waist-height. Stand facing away from the anchor, taking a handle into each hand. Bring your hands to shoulder-height with your feet staggered one in front of the other and knees slightly bent. The band should be taut in this position. Press your arms straight overhead, palms facing forward. Keep your arms as close as you can to your body as you do so.

Lower your arms back down to the starting position to finish 1 rep.

13. Cobra Pull

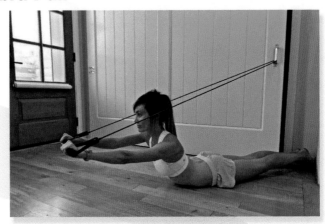

Resistance Band: Tube with Handles
Targets: Back and Shoulders

Anchor the center of your band a foot or two off of the ground (about knee height). Lie down on your stomach, head facing away from the anchor, legs together and tops of the feet on the ground. With a handle in each hand, lift your upper body off of the ground with your arms extended straight in front of you, several inches off the ground and palms down. In this position, the tube should be taut. Your hips, legs, and feet should remain on the ground throughout the entire exercise.

Return to the starting position, lying flat on your stomach and arms resting on the ground with elbows bent, before starting the next rep.

14. Standing Twist

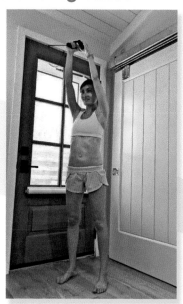
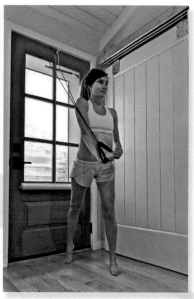

Resistance Band: Tube with Handles
Targets: Core

Secure the band at head height or higher. Stand so that your right side is facing the anchor and with your feet slightly wider than hip-width apart. Bring your hands together, holding a handle in each hand. Extend your arms straight up towards the anchor – the band should be taut in this position. Pivoting on your right foot, twist to the left side extending your arms straight across your body. With straight arms, bring both hands to your left hip.

Return to your starting position slowly. Repeat all of your reps on one side before switching sides to finish 1 set.

15. Seated Twist

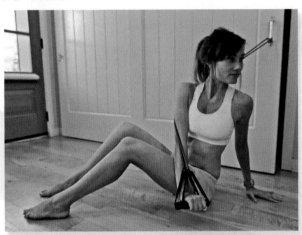

Resistance Band: Tube with Handles
Targets: Biceps, Triceps, Core, and Back

Anchor the center of the band a few feet off the ground. Sit down on the ground with knees bent and your right side facing the anchor a foot or two away. Grab both handles with the right hand, elbow bent. Twist to your left and touch your right hand to the ground by your left hip. Use your left hand as a support behind you to help keep your back straight. Make sure your feet stay on the ground throughout the exercise. Slowly twist back to the starting position.

Repeat all of your reps on 1 side before turning to sit the other way and finishing the set.

16. Muscle Beach

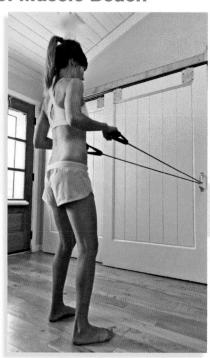 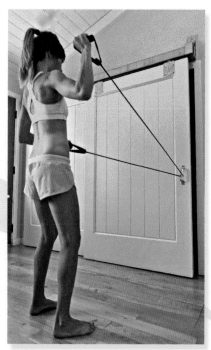

Resistance Band: Tube with Handles
Targets: Back and Shoulders

Anchor the center of the band at about chest height. Stand with your feet hip width apart and knees slightly bent. Take a handle into each hand and extend your arms straight out in front of you, palms down. Bend the elbows and pull both arms in towards your chest. Raise the elbows to the side so that your upper arms are level with the ground. Rotating from the shoulder, move the right arm so that it stays at a 90-degree angle while bringing the palm to face the anchor in front of you.

Lower that hand back to the original position and repeat with the other arm to finish 1 rep.

17. Bicep Curl Lunge

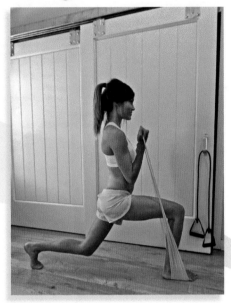

Resistance Band: Flat
Targets: Legs, Glutes, and Biceps

Stand with your feet staggered several feet apart, right foot in front. Your toes should be pointing forward and the center of the band under your right foot. Hold the ends of the band in each hand, making sure that the band is taut when your arms are straight at your side. Keeping your feet where they are, lunge forward by bending your right knee to a 90-degree angle and lowering your left knee towards the ground. As you lunge, curl your arms by bending your elbows. Bring your hands towards your chest while keeping the elbows close to the body.

Stay in the lunge position for all of the reps – complete all of your reps on one side before switching sides to finish 1 set.

18. Banded Bicycle

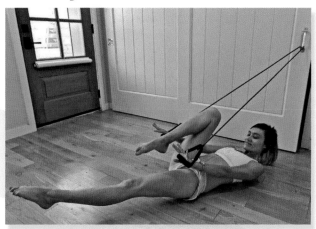

Resistance Band: Tube with Handles
Targets: Shoulders, Triceps, and Core

Find an anchor for the center of the band a few feet off of the ground. Lie down on your back facing away from the anchor with knees bent. Hold a handle in each hand. Pulse the arms down straight to your sides with palms down as you crunch up and extend one leg straight out in front of you, several inches off of the ground. As you bend the straightened leg back to the starting position, raise your arms back over your head.

Repeat with the other leg to finish 1 rep.

19. Squat Pull Down

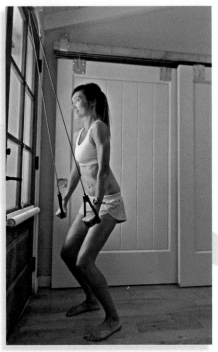

Resistance Band: Tube with Handles
Targets: Back, Glutes, and Legs

Secure the center of the tube at door-height. Stand with your feet just wider than shoulder-width apart facing the anchor. Take a handle into each hand with your arms extended straight out in front of you, palms facing down. Come into a squat, keeping the back straight and weight in your heels.

Come halfway out of the squat keeping your knees still slightly bent. As you do so, bring your arms straight at your sides, palms facing your body. This is 1 rep.

20. Triceps Press

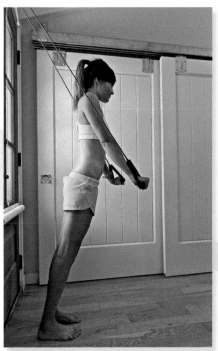

Resistance Band: Tube with Handles
Targets: Triceps

Anchor the band at door height or higher. Stand a foot or two away from the anchor with feet hip-width apart. Take a handle into each hand and bend your elbows to a 90-degree angle, palms facing down. Lean forward slightly (about 45 degrees) and press your hands down so that your arms become straight.

Slowly return your hands to the starting position to finish 1 rep.

21. Short Row

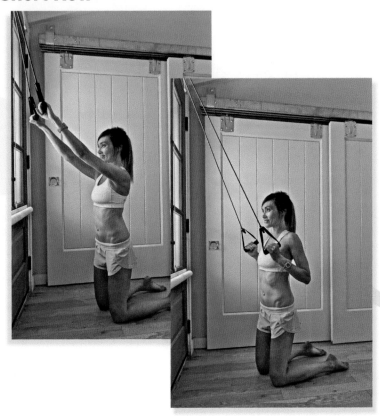

Resistance Band: Tube with Handles
Targets: Back

Secure the center of the band at door-height. Kneel a few feet away from the anchor, knees hip-width apart, facing the anchor. Take a handle into each hand. Pull down on the handles, keeping the elbows close to the body and back straight. Pull as far back as possible until the hands are at the chest. Squeeze the shoulder blades together.

Hold this position for a breath before slowly bringing your arms straight and back over your head. This is 1 rep.

22. Side Row

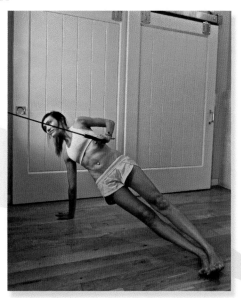

Resistance Band: Tube with Handles
Targets: Back, Core, Arms, and Shoulders

Secure one end of the tube at about knee-height. With the resistance band in your left hand come into a side plank position, placing your right hand flat on the ground directly under your shoulder and stacking the left foot on top of the right with legs straight. Your hips and legs should lift off the ground, leaving only your right hand and your right foot in contact with the floor.

Extend your left arm out in front of you level with the floor. In this position the band should be taut. Keep the elbow as close to the body as possible as you bring your left hand towards your chest. Return to the starting position to complete 1 rep.

Do all of your reps on 1 side before switching sides to finish the set.

If this version of side plank is too difficult, bring your left foot in front of you on the ground to act like a supportive "kickstand."

23. Lawn Mower

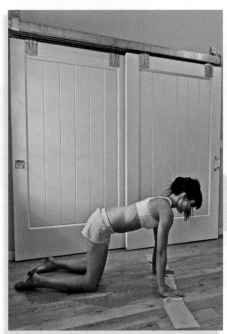 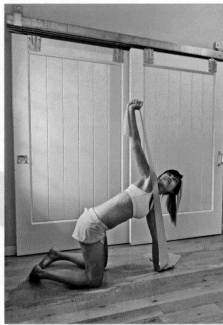

Resistance Band: Flat
Targets: Shoulders and Core

Start on all fours with your knees hip width apart. Place the band under your hands so that it is flat on the floor. Leave the left palm flat to anchor the band while you grab the band with your right hand. Keeping both arms straight, lift the right hand off the ground and rotate the torso to the right. Reach your right hand up over your head as high as possible. Slowly return to the starting position.

Do all of your reps on one side before switching sides to finish 1 set.

24. The Hundred Core

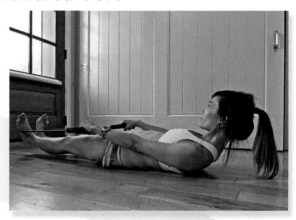

Resistance Band: Tube with Handles
Targets: Core

Lie down on your back. Place the center of the tube over your feet and grab onto the handles, one in each hand. Lift your feet about a few inches off the ground, heels together and toes apart – your legs should remain straight. Lifting your head and shoulders off of the ground, begin to pulse the arms up and down (arms straight), palms facing the ground.

Pulse the arms 50 times for 1 set. (The "hundred" comes from counting each half pulse - up and down -, but it's easier to only count each full pulse.)

25. T Lift

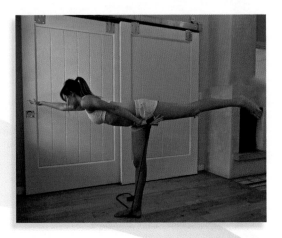

Resistance Band: Tube with Handles
Targets: Triceps, Back, Glutes, and Legs

Stand on the center of your band with your right foot acting as an anchor. Hold the handle in your left hand. As you lift your left leg up and back, straighten your right arm in front of you, in line with the ground. Reach the left arm straight back at your side, palm facing up. Keep the left leg straight, working to create one straight line from left toes to right fingertips. Slowly lower back down to the starting position.

Repeat all of your reps on one side before switching sides to complete 1 set.

26. Diagonal Toe Touch

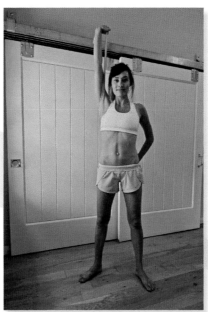

Resistance Band: Flat
Targets: Glutes, Legs, Shoulders, and Back

Hold the band behind your back. Bring your left hand to the lower back and the right hand straight up over your head. The band should be taut in this position. Stand with your feet wide and toes slightly turning out. Fold forward from the hips, bringing your right hand to the left toe. Keep the legs straight. Return to the starting position with the right arm overhead.

Do all of your reps on one side before switching sides to finish 1 set.

27. Pressing Lunge

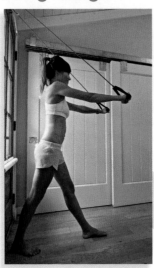 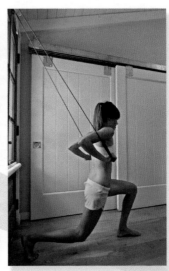

Resistance Band: Tube with Handles
Targets: Legs, Glutes, and Chest

Secure the center of the band at shoulder height or higher. Face away from the anchor and stagger your feet several feet apart, left foot forward. Hold onto the handles, one in each hand, palms facing the floor. With your legs straight, extend your arms straight out in front of you and level with the floor. As you lunge forward, bend the elbows and allow your hands to come to your chest (if the tube is no longer taut with bent elbows, make adjustments – like standing further away from the anchor – so it is). Straighten the legs and the arms to return to starting position.

Do all of your reps on one side before switching sides to finish 1 set.

28. Knockout

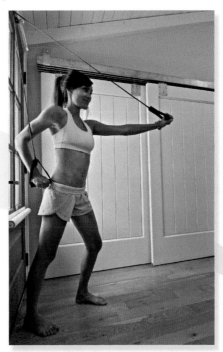

Resistance Band: Tube with Handles
Targets: Back and Core

Secure the center of the resistance band at chest height or higher. Standing with your feet hip-width apart, take a handle into each hand. Stagger your feet, left foot a few inches in front of the right. The band should be taut with your arms extended straight out in front of you. Pull the right hand to your waist, bending your elbow, and rotating your torso to that side.

Come back to center and repeat the punch on the other side to finish 1 rep.

29. Flying Warrior

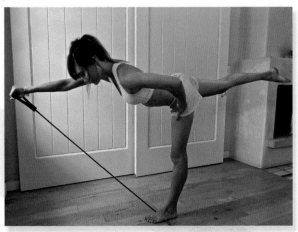

Resistance Band: Tube with Handles
Targets: Shoulders, Back, Core, Glutes, and Legs

Stand in a lunge position with your left foot anchoring the center of the tube, both knees bent. Grab the handle with your right hand, placing your left hand on your hip. Shift your weight forward into the left leg and straighten both legs, lifting the right leg into the air and the right arm straight overhead. Try to get your raised leg and arm level with the ground. Lower back to the starting position slowly.

Do all your reps on one side before switching sides to finish the set.

30. Band Press

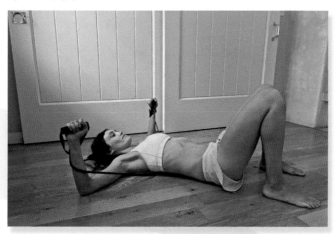

Resistance Band: Tube with Handles
Targets: Triceps and Chest

Lie on your back on top of the center of your band. Bend your knees but keep the soles of your feet on the ground. Take a handle into each of your hands with your palms facing away from you. Allow your elbows and your upper arms to rest on the ground. Press the band up as you extend your arms straight over your body, like you are doing a bench press. Adjust resistance as necessary by doubling the band or tying knots in the end so that the handles are closer to the center.

With control lower your hands back down to your chest. This is 1 rep.

EXERCISE INDEX

Triceps

- Band Wrap Push-Ups
- Triceps Raise
- Triceps Press
- Side Row
- Seated Twist
- Boxer
- Side Reach
- T Lift
- Banded Bicycle
- Band Press

Biceps

- Rows
- Bicep Curl Lunge
- Rolling Row
- High Low Pull
- Side Row
- Seated Twist
- Side Reach

Shoulders

- Squat Press
- Karate Kid
- Lawn Mower
- Diagonal Toe Touch
- Overhead Press

- Side Row
- Muscle Beach
- Boxer
- Side Reach
- Flying Warrior
- Banded Bicycle
- Cobra Pull

Back

- Rows
- Karate Kid
- Rolling Row
- Diagonal Toe Touch
- Squat Pull Down
- Side Row
- Seated Twist
- Knockout
- Short Row
- Muscle Beach
- Boxer
- Flying Warrior
- T Lift
- Cobra Pull

Chest

- Band Wrap Push-Ups
- Pressing Lunge
- Band Press

Core

- Band Wrap Push-Ups
- Standing Twist
- Lawn Mower
- Rowing Roll
- The Hundred Core
- High Low Pull
- Side Row
- Seated Twist
- Knockout
- Side Reach
- Flying Warrior
- Banded Bicycle
- Cobra Pull

Glutes

- Squat Press
- Bicep Curl Lunge
- All-Fours Donkey Kick

- Diagonal Toe Touch
- Open Close
- High Low Pull
- Pressing Lunge
- Squat Pull Down
- Flying Warrior
- T Lift

Legs

- Squat Press
- Bicep Curl Lunge
- Karate Kid
- Diagonal Toe Touch
- Open Close
- Pressing Lunge
- Squat Pull Down
- Flying Warrior
- T Lift

BONUS WORKOUT SOUNDTRACKS

Ready to pump up the jams?
Discover great soundtracks for your workouts by visiting the link below:

www.littlepearlpublishing.com/workoutjams

Discover More Great Books At

www.littlepearlpublishing.com